HYPNOTIC EROTIC

"Exceptionally well written."

Pamela A. Paradowski Ph. D.
Clinical Psychologist

"In working with thousands of individuals over the years, sexual issues are much more prevalent than they are discussed. Dr. Edgette's book is an invaluable tool for practitioners looking to offer a helpful approach. A real gem!"

Dr. Tracy Riley, LCSW
Author of "Ethical Cheating: Exploring the Swinger Lifestyle"

"**Compelling!** Hypnotic Erotic is a terrific guide to using your hypnosis skills to increase your client's sexual satisfaction. Edgette takes what can be a sensitive subject and shows you how to guide both men and women to the best sex of their lives. The book uses common, not clinical language, and Edgette provides inductions, suggestions, and even a complete script. Hypnotic Erotic is a great addition to your hypnosis tool kit!"

Dr. Linda Wells
Educator and hypnotist

"Dr. Edgette's work is groundbreaking. He explains the application of hypnotic techniques to the issues of sexual dysfunction and why these techniques readily bypass conscious defenses typically eliminating the need for patients who have to deal with powerful feelings of shame, fear, and in some instances anger. With a no nonsense approach – devoid of psychobabble – Dr. Edgette presents clear explanations of powerful proven hypnotic techniques and applies them in uniquely novel ways designed specifically to alleviate the many varieties of sexual dysfunction.

Any therapist treating patients suffering from sexual dysfunction would do well to read Dr. Edgette's work."

Dr. Bill Neely
Clinical Psychologist, author of the Forthcoming book
"Patriarchy: Why the World is Fucked Up"

HYPNOTIC EROTIC:

A PRACTITIONER'S GUIDE TO
SEXUAL HEALING

Dr. John H. Edgette

John@edgettetherapy.com

Other books by Dr. John H. Edgette:

The Handbook of Hypnotic Phenomena in Psychotherapy (with J.S. Edgette)

Winning the Mind Game: Hypnosis and Sport Psychology (with Tim Rowan)

Paperback ISBN: 978-1-7354802-1-3

Published by: J. Galt & Associates

Dr. John H. Edgette
P.O. Box 1271
Fairfield, Iowa
USA
1 917-806-1850
John@edgettetherapy.com

First Printing: August 2020

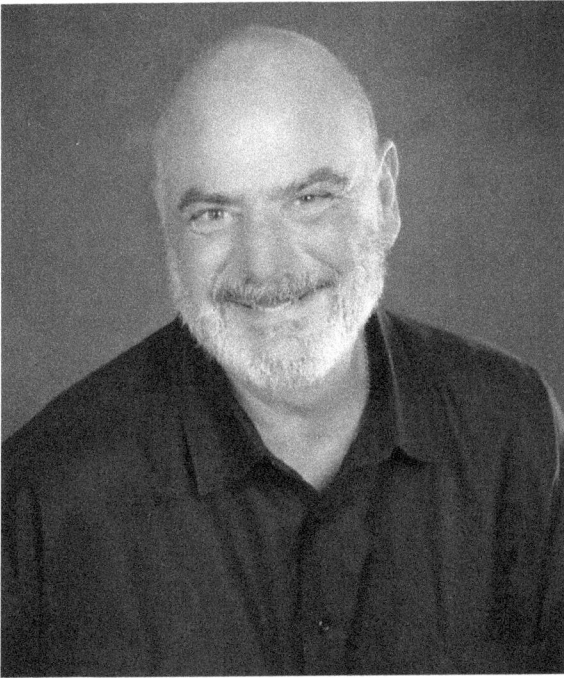

Dr. John H. Edgette received his doctoral degree in clinical psychology in 1985 from Hahnemann Medical College and Graduate School in Philadelphia, PA. He had practiced as a psychotherapist for over 30 years in agencies, clinics, group practices, and private practice.

Now practicing as a sexologist, life coach, and certified hypnosis consultant, he was licensed as a clinical psychologist in Iowa, Illinois, and Pennsylvania. He is the author of 3 books and over 7 journal articles. His

I

works have been translated into 7 languages. He has been asked to give keynote addresses and seminars at over 50 professional conferences and has taught in over 30 states and 15 countries around the world.

As America's foremost hypnosis "sex-pert", John is the first Dr. of clinical psychology to affirm that kink, fetish, BDSM, Dom/sub, and swinging can be healthy for couples and even enhance intimacy in relationships.

LGBTQ++ friendly and a sex positive feminist, he is prominently listed in the directory "Kink Aware Professionals" which is hosted by The National Coalition for Sexual Freedom.

Dr. John Edgette is available to practitioners via Zoom or FaceTime for individual consultations and advice regarding clients with sexuality or other issues. He is also available for sessions with any individual having issues with sexuality or a variety of other problems.

For more information call, text, e-mail, or FaceTime him (see the contact info)

To Dr. Alfred Kinsey, my mentor in absentia.

I

TABLE OF CONTENTS

PART ONE: FOREPLAY

Dr. John H. Edgette

CHAPTER 1
Introduction:

"I am a total fucking failure." Jimbo had emailed me requesting a tele-hypnosis session to fix a "small" problem. "Even though I take Viagra I still can't get it up!" he gushed out.

In the first session, where I got to know Jimbo and learned about his issue, I did an initial hypnotic induction with him. He was a very good subject so in that, and a subsequent session, I cultivated his ability to produce the hypnotic phenomena of arm levitation, complete with the classic qualities of his arm being stiff, rigid, and feeling like wood.

In the third and final session I connected those qualities to his member and gave him the post-hypnotic suggestion to re-experience it whenever he wanted to have sex. I simply said "let your arm now lower and come to rest on your dick. All the feelings in your arm can transfer to your cock as if a water faucet had opened and now it all flows into your male meat and you can have this experience anytime you wish simply by remembering this transfer vividly and fully."

There was to be a fourth session but he cancelled it. "Doc, I'm fixed!" he exclaimed.

Hypnosis is the ideal way to resolve sexual problems, quickly. This is because influencing the subconscious mind is the fastest and most effective way to change how sexuality is expressed.

This book will give you all the tools you need to create sexual solutions using hypnosis. So read on, learn how to heal current clients while developing a

whole new specialty that attracts an underserved population!

This book was written because there was a total absence of any good information on this topic. Anything that does exist is either authoritarian in tone or downright hokey in nature. For example "Your penis will be hard as a rock or a steel girder for hours on end."

In addition, this book is **different** because it is written from a sex positive feminist philosophical orientation. Also, it employs the pioneering model of hypnosis developed by Milton H. Erickson M.D. The work contained within is collaborative, permissive, resource eliciting and solution finding. Moreover, it is **unique** in being the only book of its kind written by a professional.

The tone of this book is very **liberal**. I believe that as long as acts are safe, sane, and consensual, they can be engaged in without guilt. Also, the sexual language used is visceral, candid, guttural, and graphic. I don't believe that effective sexual healing can take place by using sterile and sanitary words like penis, vagina, fellatio, and cunnilingus. Who wants that? Everyone would rather have a cock, a pussy, and give a blow job or go down on a woman. These terms are therapeutic, while the use of "proper" terms are either ineffective or counterproductive in their hygienic nature. As writer Elmore Leonard said, "If it sounds like writing, I rewrite it. Or, if proper usage gets in the way, it may have to go. I can't allow what we learned in English composition to disrupt the sound and rhythm of the narrative."

The first part of this book will **refresh** one's knowledge of how to put a person into trance and how to give suggestions in hypnosis. These chapters will also serve the person **learning** hypnosis for the first time. After those initial chapters the reader will be taught (or reminded of) how to use an array of hypnotic phenomena for change. These subconscious capabilities are essential for intervening with sexual issues. In that regard they complement the use of direct suggestion or metaphors to solicit change. Readers learning the above for the initial time may want to supplement the chapters in this book with live training or introductory books.

After the first section of this book, the rest of the book is devoted to teaching the reader how to relieve various sexual issues quickly, competently, and effectively. These chapters are succinct yet comprehensive.

Hypnosis is the fastest way to resolve sexual problems and this book will teach you all you will need to do that. So, come on and read on!

CHAPTER 2
Induction Method # 1: Double Binds

First off, as a reminder, the chapters that follow are designed for those who once learned hypnosis and are in need of a refresher or those who are learning for the first time. If you fall into the latter category it would be a good idea to supplement what you find here with additional reading, live teaching, and some one-on-one consulting with a very experienced practitioner. In the meantime, readers are most welcome to e-mail me with any questions.

Hypnotizing someone is incredibly easy. Hypnotizing someone else so that they can hypnotize themselves is easier still, and the easiest of all is to hypnotize yourself. Whether you are in this to entrance your client, help your client entrance themselves, or put yourself under, the procedures in the following "Foreplay" chapters, taken as a whole, accomplish that mission.

Hypnosis has often been made to seem very hard, technical, mysterious, and requiring incredible precision. There are probably at least three reasons for this: one reason is so that students are held in constant awe and confusion and continue to pay high prices for multitudes of courses. The second reason may be that the teachers wish to see themselves as very advanced, educated, scientific, and wise, and desire to have their students see them in the same way. A third reason may be that there is then a greater placebo effect from the use of hypnosis as a procedure.

Yet simple it remains.

Dr. John H. Edgette

To start, find out from your subject what they have heard or experienced about hypnosis. Affirm the validity of all reports describing how hypnosis was a very helpful tool in enlisting the aid of the subconscious mind in overcoming a problem such as an addiction or pain. If the client cites anything that they worry about in connection with hypnosis, assure them with confidence that this is an unneeded worry. *There is absolutely no loss of control in hypnosis. People cannot be made to do anything that they do not want to do while in trance. People come out of hypnosis whenever they please. The worst thing that can happen in hypnosis is that nothing happens.*

To begin the actual hypnosis, employ this first induction strategy. As a prelude though, have the client sit comfortably in a chair, in a sustainable position, muscles relaxed, eyes closed. Assure them that there is nothing they need to do, that you will do all of the work, and that their unconscious will respond accordingly.

Then begin the double bind induction. Find a sample outline below. Be sure to use permissive language, that is; "you will" should be avoided in favor of "you may, or "you can". People generally don't like to be told what to do. People prefer having their ability to choose validated and not challenged.

This double bind induction is also referred to as the "illusion of alternatives" because it offers a choice between two alternatives, both of which are desirable for the creation and experience of trance.

Say phrases like the following:

- "You can go into hypnosis quickly or slowly."
- "You may develop a light trance or a deep trance."
- "You can allow yourself to drift into trance listening to the sound of my voice or to the sounds in the room."
- "Perhaps you will begin to notice a lightness or maybe a comfortable heaviness as you flow down into hypnosis."
- "You can move forward into trance by opening up to the creative possibilities inherent in

hypnosis or you can focus on re-connecting with your own personal history of success."

After you are done saying these slowly, with a deep voice, then you can repeat the phrases once or twice or better yet, make up more of your own. After that you can utilize another type of induction, which you will find in the chapters that follow.

CHAPTER 3
Induction Method # 2
Conscious – Unconscious
Dissociative Statements

Healthy, natural and productive dissociation is the hallmark of being hypnotised. To foster dissociation in service of "creating trance" you can verbally separate the conscious and subconscious parts of the mind via the sentences below. Say them in order or randomly. Invent your own too. After you are done you can repeat or go back to induction method #1 or onto the methods that follow. However, if the client is hypnotised then you can proceed to the intervention stage of trance work. As before, if this induction is being used for self-hypnosis it is best that it is audio taped as it is far too hard to think about what to say and still go into trance.

Conscious – Unconscious Dissociative Statements

Your Conscious Mind	Causal Link	Your Unconscious Mind
1. Is listening to my words	And	Is doing something else
2. May be interested in learning one thing	And	Is concerned with what's relevant
3. May have certain doubts	While	Understands and absorbs what you need
4. Is very linear	While	Can provide you with a mosaic of creative potentials
5. Intellectualizes, analyzes, and compartmentalizes	Just as	It is an infinite storehouse of talents, learnings and possibilities
6. May be easily diverted	Because	Can allow things to happen in your own best interest

CHAPTER 4
Hypnotic Induction Method 3-
ABC and 1, 2, 3

This induction method consists of an age regression back in time to metaphorically teach the subject how to reconnect to past resources. By doing so the client goes into trance as part of regressing. This induction accomplishes two things at once: entrancing the subject while also prepping them for the intervention phase of hypnosis by giving them an object lesson in resource retrieval (learning that they can learn to do something that appears horridly difficult at first).

While the hypnotist can read this script verbatim, feel free to be creative and riff off of it. Again, after saying this if the client is not in trance use methods #1 and #2 or method #4 which follows. Also, if this is to be used for autohypnosis it is best to tape the induction.

This induction is a transcript of the actual work of the pioneering legendary hypnotist Milton Erickson M.D. His grammar, syntax, and usage has been preserved as spoken for accuracy of intent.

"And I'm going to talk about something that occurred in your childhood when you first went to school and had to learn to write the letters of the alphabet. It seemed like a terribly difficult task. All those letters, all those different shapes. Do you dot the "e, i" and cross the "i"? And where do you put the loop on the "b" and the "d" and the "p"? And how many bumps on the letter "m"? Gradually you formed a mental image of each letter, many mental images, because letters are in script and in print various shapes and sizes and finally you had mental images located somewhere in your brain and you added mental images of persons and words and numbers and objects and even ideas. Not knowing at the time you were forming mental images.

While I've been talking to you your respiration has changed, your blood pressure has changed. Your muscle tone has changed and your muscle reflexes have changed. Close your eyes now and feel the sense of comfort. The more comfortable you feel the deeper into a trance you'll go.

In the trance state you can let your unconscious mind (pause) survey that vast array of learnings that you achieve, that you have achieved during your lifetime. There are many learnings that you've made without knowing it. Many of the learnings that were very important to you consciously have slipped into your unconscious mind and have become automatically useful to you and are used only at the right time, in the right situation.

Learning to walk was a very difficult task but you achieved it. Now you don't know just exactly how you walk down the street, how you move your feet and your legs, your arms, move your head, how far from the curb you slow down, what buildings you veer toward and what buildings you veer away from. You don't know which way you first move your head when you first reach an intersection. But you will look to the right and to the left and ahead. You'll make a lot of movements. You'll make a lot of movements even if there is no traffic of any kind.

When you first learned to drive a car that was a very big task to put on the brakes and stop at the intersection when you are traveling 10 miles an hour. But as you became an expert driver you could see a stop sign in the distance and it didn't make a bit of difference whether you were traveling 70, 60, 50, 40, 30 miles an hour. At the right time, at the right distance, with the right degree of force you applied the brake and rolled to a gentle stop. You don't even know how you measured that distance. You don't know what sense of body movement entered into it; what your peripheral vision told you and now I could sit in the back seat of the car you are driving and I would know at least a half a block in advance when you were going to turn right or left by your body language. I might know it even before you realize, "Oh, here's the street I turn on."

Your unconscious mind knows much more than you do. Your conscious mind has an awareness and it's oriented to the situation of the moment and so you're aware of desks and bookcases, wall hangings, telephone, which have nothing to do with your purpose in coming. But your unconscious mind can disregard all those irrelevant facts and pay attention to my words and pay attention to its own reactions."

> *Reprinted from…*
> THE ANSWER WITHIN:
> A Clinical Framework of
> Ericksonian Hypnotherapy
> By Lankton & Lankton 1983

CHAPTER 5
The Three-Sentence Induction Method #4

This induction consists of three simple sentences that when verbalised puts a client into trance, it is easy to remember and replicate so there is never a need to tape, but of course you always can. As always, this induction can stand alone or be combined with the other three or even ones you have learned elsewhere. It was developed by G. Andrewartha.

In preparing for the Three-Sentence Induction, clients are given the following directions:

1. Explain to the subject you are going to use a very simple process of trance induction.

2. Have the subject sit comfortably with their feet resting on the floor, and their arms placed comfortably in their lap.

3. Commence the induction with sentence one.

Use a lower voice tone where indicated and develop a repetitive rhythm. The sentences are as follows:

1. You may allow (pause) what you are experiencing right now (pause) just to continue.

2. You may be really curious (pause) about just how comfortable (pause) you can be.

3. It's not necessary for you (pause) to go deeply into trance.

The first sentence effectively introduces the induction, gives permission, aids rapport, and matches the subject's experience. The subject need only to continue doing whatever he or she is doing to be behaving appropriately.

The second sentence reinforces many of the elements of the first. The words "really curious" also introduce elements of drama and expectation, as well as age regression.

The third sentence utilizes potential resistance or noncompliance. It incorporates the embedded command "go deeply into trance." This also contains a double bind, so a subject who chooses not to go deeply into trance may, implicitly, go lightly into trance.

By their nature and repetition, the sentences have proven to foster amnesia, time distortion, and dissociation. Once trance is established, these sentences also deepen the trance experience.

The use of this technique can result in the induction of a moderate-to-deep trance in 15 minutes or as rapidly as 1 minute.

CHAPTER 6
Ratification and Deepening

After induction the next step in hypnotizing is ratification. I am either reminding you of this or teaching you this for the first time. Regardless, here is a succinct and efficient protocol for ratifying trance.

First though, let's define ratification. Ratification is the act of verbally stating or feeding back to the client that which you observe is indicative of trance.

The purpose of ratification is to notify the client that he or she is cooperating by going into hypnosis. To this end you name the indicators or markers of hypnotic involvement that you observe. This serves an educational purpose in stating what they are doing correctly. In effect, you are telling them what to do more of so they can go deeper into hypnosis. Another reason to ratify is to provide a social reinforcement; by telling them what you see is indicative of trance you are telling them in effect that they are doing the right thing. This serves as a positive social reinforcement, as does the implication that they are pleasing you, the hypnotist. A final reason to ratify is to train your eye to notice trance indicators. The more you observe the more you know, with regard, to how well you are hypnotizing and most importantly, how well you are hypnotizing this particular client. In summary, by ratifying you educate and train the client and yourself by providing observations and reinforcements with the end result that you hypnotize more effectively and the client gets hypnotized more efficiently.

Here is a list of things you might look for when ratifying:

- Very slow body movements
- Eventually, no body movement unless suggested (naturally occurring catalepsy)

- Ever deeper and slower breathing
- Pulse slows
- Muscles become very relaxed
- Head drooping
- Body tilting and becoming more asymmetrical
- Jaw slackening
- Upon awakening a greatly distorted sense of how much time has passed (ask)
- Upon reorienting reports having had feelings of dissociation
- Reports a quiet, silent mind

This is not an exhaustive list. Nonetheless, after your inductions, start feeding back to your client the things which you see them manifesting from the above list. As Milton Erickson would say, "observe, observe, observe".

As I would say:

"I can see you are going into hypnosis because your breath rate has slowed, your heart rate has slowed, and your muscles look very, very relaxed."

"I know that you're going down into trance because your head can't help itself from dropping down, your body is tilting off to one side and you probably don't even know it yet, or if you do you don't care. Also, your jaw is getting relaxed so your mouth is now open and you are even drooling a little bit. Don't worry about that, if it gets worse I will put a lobster bib on you (no laughter, people lose their sense of humor in hypnosis).

The conversation upon awakening: "How much time do you think passed?" "Fifteen minutes, no, probably 10." "It was actually 45 minutes...... you were deep in trance. This is proof that people can't tell time in hypnosis."

Ratification tends to initially bring a person out of trance because the conscious mind gets focused and evaluative causing some beta wave brain activity and hence a bit of "fight or flight" sympathetic nervous system arousal. Yet on the heels of that the subconscious mind takes over and relaxes again, and the person actually winds up going deeper into trance. So ratification is actually a method of deepening as well as helping one to attain the other hypnotic goals above.

In general, when a person goes in and out of hypnosis it deepens the trance. This is called "fractionation". It is one of the most powerful methods of deepening. You can effect this by ratifying or by simply bringing a person out of hypnosis repeatedly and then putting the person back in.

You know you need to deepen if you do not see many signs of trance to ratify.

The simplest way to deepen, easier than using fractionation, is to simply use more inductions. Do as many as you need to until you see multiple signs of hypnosis taking place, such as when you can easily note them aloud to effect ratification.

The above, I trust, you can figure out but to bring a person in and out of trance you would say something like this: "You can bring yourself a bit out of trance either going to a later stage of hypnosis or coming all the way out. If you come all the way out you open your eyes

27

and look at me and then immediately you'll go back down into an even deeper state of hypnosis that you have achieved previously here or anywhere else."

So that is how you ratify and deepen. Do it after your induction. Have at it!

CHAPTER 7
The Art of Giving Self Suggestion

Much attention has been given to the topic of self-hypnosis, both for adults and for children. When the topic of giving oneself suggestions, in hypnosis, is addressed it is almost always as if it is simply a matter of saying words to oneself, once the induction has been completed. This approach limits the potential for effective self -suggestion because it frames the intervention as being linguistic and technical only. Having the proper mental stance or attitudinal position is, at least, as important as the words themselves.

I propose a set of illustrative metaphors that will enable the practitioner, child or adult, of self -hypnosis to adopt an optimal psychological position vis-à-vis the suggestion being given such that it has maximum effect.

These metaphors harken to times in the past where the optimal mental attitude was present. As such, they provide a historical reference point and resource for the practitioner of self- hypnosis so that they can easily adopt a proper psychological position that will enable the desired suggestion to have maximum impact.

Please note that these illustrative metaphors are appropriate for all but the stodgiest adults. That is to say, no doubt there are some CPAs, engineers, and surgeons, who will balk at their playful and often regressive nature. Nonetheless, for most, they will serve as an ideal template with which to understand what is meant by an optimal mental attitude or stance.

Self-suggestions are best conceived as personal wishes embedded in an optimal psychological framework. The wish alone is not enough, it must be put forth coming out of the right attitude that will enable the self that the wishes be fulfilled.

The following metaphors will quickly serve to show subjects the correct way to wish their self-hypnotic wishes:

- "Everyone has had the experience of being presented with a birthday cake with candles on it. Your task then becomes to take a moment and make a wish for something to come true while seeking to blow out all the candles so that it does."

- "Many of us have seen a shooting star in the night sky. When we do, we quickly make a wish in the hopes that viewing this phenomena will allow it to come true."

- "More commonly, all of us have seen the first star in the night sky. At that moment, we take the opportunity to offer up a wish that we hope will take place."

- "On Thanksgiving Day it is common for a dried out turkey wishbone to be grabbed at each end by two small children who then pull each end and break it. The one who gets the bigger piece either makes a wish on the spot, which he/she hopes to come true, or hopes that the wish that he made prior to the contest comes to fruition."

- "Just about every one of us has had the opportunity to throw a coin into a fountain or a pool of water. Prior to tossing the coin you make a wish and then upon tossing the coin gently, hope that it will come true."

These metaphors are common everyday examples, many from childhood, that adeptly illustrate the optimal mental approach or attitude to giving oneself wishes or self-suggestions. We all secretly recognize that what we are hoping for is some shift in conscious or subconscious functioning, such that the environment reacts differently to us and our wish comes to fruition. It is the law of attraction.

Since all hypnosis is self- hypnosis, the psychological positioning's illustrated above can be utilized in hetero hypnosis.

Please note that some of these metaphors may be culturally bound. Obviously, if the metaphor is not found in a particular culture it makes little sense to use it, unless you are enchanting a person with possibilities that exist in other cultures.

When working in non-North American cultures, it can be interesting and useful to find out the contexts within which wishes are seen to actualize. I can remember asking about this while teaching in Russia, there were many very interesting and unique examples of times when wishes might easily come to fruition. One that stands in mind concerns the notion that if a person is standing between two people of the same name it is lucky. Therefore, it is a superb time to make a wish for something you want to come true. That is to say if you have a man named Andre on your right and another man named Andre on your left you have satisfied the conditions for good fortune with regard to any wish made.

It is my hope that this approach to making self-suggestion will increase the effectiveness of these wishes

Dr. John H. Edgette

for change. Such is been my experience in clinical practice and I think it makes good clinical sense that hypnotic suggestions to oneself should be more than just a set of words introduced after an induction.

For those wishing to learn more about giving self-suggestions, read Dr. Richard Nongard's book on the topic entitled "

CHAPTER 8
What Are Hypnotic Phenomena And How Do I Use Them?

As you will see in the various chapters in this book, hypnotic phenomena are incredibly useful in resolving sexual issues. Here they are defined and described.

Hypnotic phenomena can be described as natural behavioral and experiential manifestations of the trance state. They include both subjectively experienced psychological events, such as remembering, forgetting, distortions in one's sense of time, and alterations in perception, as well as observable events, such as the levitation of an arm or the automatic, unconsciously driven scribbling of words across a pad.

VARIETIES OF HYPNOTIC PHENOMENA

Catalepsy is a special state of muscle tone and balance that permits the subject to sustain postures and positions for unusually long periods of time, without appreciable fatigue. It is accompanied by slowing down of all psychomotor activity and is the basis for other phenomena such as arm levitation.

An alteration in one's sense of time is another hypnotic phenomenon that is commonly experienced by subjects even under conditions of light trance. Time becomes very subjective and dissociated from standard measures. A person in trance for 25 minutes, who thinks the trance has been only 10 minutes long, is experiencing time contraction. Someone who feels a 10-minute trance to be of half an hour in duration, experiences time expansion.

Dissociation is one of the more widely recognized and experienced hypnotic phenomenas. It is a separation of psychological states into conscious and unconscious, or a separation of emotions from thoughts, behaviors, and feelings. Dissociation may also be defined as "a mental process in which systems of ideas are split off from the normal personality and operate independently". Dissociation, apart from being a vehicle of intervention in its own right, is also the process by which the development of other hypnotic phenomena, such as age regression, automatic writing, pain control, and therapeutic hallucinations, take place. After all, it is the suspension of logical, rational, and intellectualized thoughts that allow these other, seemingly irrational or regressive, experiences to be brought forth into consciousness.

Amnesia refers to a functional loss of the ability to recall or identify past experiences. It manifests, in its ability, to have subjects forget things that are generally considered impossible to forget, such as one's name and age. Amnesia can be induced in hypnosis either to ablate memories (of experience, affect, or cognition) that

37

occurred prior to the trance or ablate those being created during the trance experience itself.

Hypermnesia refers to an enhanced memory ability that transcends everyday recollection. This hypnotic phenomenon allows subjects to vividly remember memories in all their sensory detail.

The phenomenon of **age regression** is partly based upon the mechanisms of amnesia and hypermnesia. In the context of hypnosis, age regression allows one to re-experience memories of an earlier period. Age regressions differ from simple hypermnesia, in that, the subject relives rather than just remembers past events and, at times, experiences a return to the psychological state as it existed then. Thus, an adult can respond to suggestions to have amnesia for his or her adult years and return to the cognitive, affective, and behavioral experience of being a teenager. True age regressions like that, where there is a demonstrable suspension of adult faculties and motor responses, are more difficult to elicit than regressions where the subject retains adult faculties and behaviors, and simply re-experiences an earlier time/memory.

Future progression (also referred to as **age progression, future orientation** and pseudo-orientation in time) is the hypnotic phenomenon that disorients the subject away from the present and into the future. The experience can be one of seeing the future self, talking to the future self, or being the future self, with access to the imagined thoughts and feelings of the older self.

Negative and positive hallucinations refer to alterations in the subject's experience of sensory stimuli. Hallucinations can involve any of the sensory systems of vision, hearing, taste, touch, and smell. Negative hallucinations refer to the person not perceiving a stimulus that actually does exist in the immediate environment. For instance, a person who is sensitive to cigarette odor and who works in an environment where smoking is present may be helped to reduce her perception of cigarette smoke in the air via negative olfactory hallucinations. A teenager taunted at school can learn to effect negative auditory hallucinations for the comments of his pesky or cruel peers. A sales manager anxious about giving an oral report to a roomful of supervisors can use negative visual hallucinations to blur the clarity with which she recognizes their faces.

Hypnotic blindness, color blindness, and **deafness** (extremes of the phenomenon of negative hallucination) have been reported. This ability of the body to ignore the perception of specific sensory stimuli is one of the bases for using anesthesia and analgesia for pain control.

Positive hallucinations refer to a person's experience of a sensory stimulus that is not actually present. Thus, a person can use the positive olfactory hallucination of liniment as a post-hypnotic cue to gear up for an athletic competition. Positive auditory hallucinations can help a self-doubting, novice therapist recall the encouraging words of a respected supervisor or the positive feedback from a satisfied client. That same sales manager, anxious about her oral report can, alternately, be helped to create a positive visual hallucination vis-à-vis her audience of supervisors, wherein she experiences the room filled instead with family and friends or even strangers.

Automatic writing is a hypnotic phenomenon that is an outgrowth of a dissociation between conscious and unconscious mental functioning. The subject, in response to direct or indirect suggestions to write, does in fact write with pen and paper but without conscious awareness, vigilance, or interference. The material may include previously repressed ideas or memories useful in propelling the client toward health. It may give rise to associations that the client then applies toward the problem resolution, or it may provide a new perspective on the problem or a solution. Also, the process of uncensored writing may actually turn out to be the most important aspect of the experience, allowing for re-engagement with a more liberated, creative, and disinhibited part of the self. **Automatic drawing** or **painting** would be, of course, the artistic correlates to automatic writing.

Posthypnotic suggestion refers to the execution, at some later (post-trance) time or date, of instructions or suggestions given during trance. A couple using hypnosis for childbirth can be told together in trance that their first sighting of the hospital when they drive up during labor will automatically begin the upper/lower body dissociation and anesthesia sensations practiced previously in session.

Analgesia refers to a dulling in one's awareness of pain whereas **anesthesia** refers to a complete lack of awareness of pain. These hypnotic phenomena are especially useful in pain control cases where medication is contraindicated (i.e., risk of allergic reaction, or a history of drug addiction and/or abuse) or is unavailable. Pain is often a part of many sexual problems.

Hyperesthesia refers to an enhanced sensitivity to physical sensations such as touch, warmth, or coolness. Pain is not a fixed response to a painful stimulus but rather a sensation, the perception of which is modified by past experiences, expectation, and cultural attitudes. This idea provides the essential underpinnings for the viability and applicability of pain control measures such as analgesia, anesthesia, and hyperesthesia.

Hypnotic dreaming entails the subject's capacity to have, either in session or at home during sleep, a directed therapeutic dream that is an immediate by-product of the suggestion given during the session.

Ideomotor movement involves the body's motor system reacting and acting as if directed by the unconscious mind, with the result that the person feels the movement to be avolitional, that is, that the conscious mind is a passive observer. Arm levitation is one example of ideomotor movement.

Hypnotic phenomena are critical to resolving sexual problems. Their use is suggested in just about every chapter. The following chapter describes how to elicit and produce hypnotic phenomena in trance work.

DOING IT: HYPNOTIC PHENOMENA

At this point it's important that we elucidate a specific protocol through which hypnotic phenomena can be elicited. The phenomena protocol is as follows:

1. Seeding
2. Language-based suggestions for the phenomena
   a. Presuppositions
   b. Direct suggestion
   c. Double binds
   d. Conscious/subconscious dissociated statements
3. Metaphors
4. Natural examples from everyday life
5. Symbols
6. Follow-through

1. Seeding

The first thing a sexologist using hypnosis to elicit hypnotic phenomena can do is seed the hypnotic phenomena. Seeding is the hypnotic equivalent of the literary device of foreshadowing. In seeding, you hint at what is to come in the hypnosis proper. Seed prior to the actual hypnotic session and the hypnotic intervention as a way of "priming the pump".

Examples of this method are as follows:

i.   Become very curious about what kind of delightfully disarming experience you'll have in trance today. (Arm levitation)

ii. As you settle into a comfortable trance depth, your unconscious mind can begin to draw its own conclusions about the matter at hand. (Automatic drawing)

iii.   Wasn't it easy for you to have lost awareness of the traffic sounds outside? Go ahead and override the needs of your conscious mind to realize everything and let your unconscious teach **you about the beauty and simplicity of absence. (Negative hallucination)**

2. Language-based suggestions

In the hypnotic work proper there are four major language-based ways of eliciting hypnotic phenomena. First, the therapist can use pre-suppositions. Pre-suppositions constitute therapeutic assuming. Here you assume that something is going to happen and therefore the subject believes accordingly. It is an indirect way of getting the client to believe that something is true. In so expecting what they will experience.

Examples of this method are as follows:

i. Your first inkling that a dream is about to take place can be your cue to go ever more deeply into trance. (Hypnotic dreaming)

ii. Once you recognize your perception of time/space/sensation beginning to alter, your unconscious self can begin to speculate about how best to apply that different and special experience of the world. (Time distortion/dissociation positive and negative hallucination)

iii. When you first wonder whether it is warmth or numbness you feel in your hands, you can smile with pride at how well your body responds to hypnosis. (Catalepsy)

A second language-based way of noticing hypnotic phenomena is direct suggestion. This is the easiest and most obvious method of eliciting hypnotic phenomena, in that you simply and forthrightly suggest it.

Examples of this method are as follows:

i.   Invite that whimsical part of you to lift your hand — let it enchant you! (Arm levitation)

ii.   Slowly, ever so slowly, slow down inside and let time follow. (Time distortion)

iii. You, too, can be this imaginary great erotic lover right here, as a grown-up, whether or not you had one or more imaginary friends as a child. Why not ask your unconscious mind to open up those memory stores and show you again how easy it is to drum up whomever you need. (Positive visual/auditory hallucination)

Double binds constitute the third language-based way in which hypnotic phenomena can be elicited. With double binds you offer an illusion of alternatives. After you have offered such, the client feels a freedom to choose from what you've presented; two possibilities, either of which moves the client in the desired direction.

Examples of this method are as follows:

i. Perhaps it will be your left hand that begins to feel light and rise up or maybe it will be your right hand that will feel an increased sense of levity.

ii. You can develop a deep, profound, and robust amnesia for any bad putt that rattles you immediately after you make that putt, or you can develop that immense and unreachable amnesia the minute you go to make your next putt.

Conscious/subconscious dissociative statements are the fourth and final language-based way in which hypnotic phenomena can be elicited. With these suggestions the client's conscious mind is coaxed to do one productive thing related to a hypnotic phenomenon while her subconscious mind is simultaneously coaxed into doing something complementary, yet different.

Examples of this method are as follows:

i. Your conscious mind can let go of certain fragments of thoughts while your unconscious mind lets go of entire texts of ideas. (Amnesia)

ii.   Your conscious mind can become aware of feeling wistful while your unconscious mind tenderly reveals old thoughts that have some bearing on the things we spoke about today. (Hypermnesia)

3. Metaphors

Metaphors are often very helpful in eliciting hypnotic phenomena. A metaphor in our context is a story or anecdote that contains, within it, suggestions for the development of the hypnotic phenomenon in question.

Examples of sample metaphors designed to induce a specific hypnotic phenomena are as follows:

i.   Fog lifting, re-assembly of jigsaw puzzles, a series of knots being untied one by one. (Hypermnesia)

ii.   Circuit breaker, dials, "thick skin". (Anesthesia/analgesia) iii.　　Clocks with worn-out batteries, cuckoo clocks with worn-out mechanisms, daylight savings time, running through water. (Time expansion)

4. Natural examples

Natural examples of a hypnosis-like or pseudo-hypnotic nature drawn from everyday life constitute still yet another wonderful way of eliciting hypnotic phenomena. They illustrate the hypnosis that occurs in ordinary life and as such they can show people that the hypnotic phenomena we're seeking to create are not very unusual, but are in fact sometimes part and parcel of our day. While using natural examples, subjects get the sense that they are not producing something alien but instead something familiar.

Examples of natural hypnosis-like situations that can elicit hypnotic phenomena are as follows:

i.　　Szechwan chicken, hot salsa, new shoes, professional perfume developers. (Hyperesthesia)

ii. Physiological habituation to sound/temperature, absorption in a movie to the exclusion of hearing the telephone ring. (Negative hallucination)

iii. The childhood game of red light/green light, Simon Says, sprinters at the block, divers poised at the 10-meter board. (Catalepsy)

5. Symbols

Therapists can use symbols to elicit hypnotic phenomena. When you use a symbol, you are using a living representation of the hypnotic phenomenon in question.

Examples of symbols that can be developed in hypnosis to elicit a hypnotic phenomenon are as follows:

i. Mannequin (Arm levitation)

ii. Elephant toy (Hypermnesia)

iii. Etch-A-Sketch (Automatic drawing)

iv. Polygraph (Automatic writing)

v. Nursery rhyme (Age regression)

6. Follow-through

After making these suggestions designed to produce hypnotic phenomena, it's useful to follow through. Following through is as important in any athletic act as it is in hypnotic work. Therefore, after the hypnosis proper is over it is useful to mention things that will help to consolidate the intervention that was promoted during the session.

Examples of this method are as follows:

i.   Repeat what was said during the hypnosis.

ii.   Say it in a different way.

iii.   Give post-hypnotic suggestions to enable the effect to be re-experienced later.

iv.   Make verbal and visual bridges between what occurred in hypnosis and everyday life.

v.   Ask the client how she thinks she might use the intervention just suggested in the hypnotic session.

Sometime after eliciting the hypnotic phenomena for intervention, but before following through, be sure to connect what you have produced to the sexual problem at hand. In other words, after you have elicited catalepsy for example, attach that solution to the client's issue. For eg. "Now that your arm is erect, rigid, still, and a bit numb, you are welcome to intermittently, as needed, experience this when you have sex and you won't come early, you will last." That connection seals the deal!

For more information on hypnotic phenomena and how to produce it, read my book "The Handbook of Hypnotic Phenomena in Psychotherapy" (by Dr. John H. Edgette).

CHAPTER 9
De-hypnotizing Your Client

Bringing your client out of hypnosis is ridiculously easy. Simply tell them to come out of hypnosis. Yup, that is right! Example of what to say is at the end of this chapter.

While anyone can be hypnotized, if they want to be hypnotized, no one can be hypnotized if they don't want to be. What this means is that no one is "**UNDER YOUR CONTROL**", or mine, thank goodness. I sure don't want that responsibility! What that also means is that anyone can come out of hypnosis if they wish to.

Moreover, research has shown that if no suggestions are given for ending the trance then almost everyone automatically comes out on their own in minutes. So even if you remain silent or even leave the room, things will work out just fine! Anyone that does not come out of hypnosis is making an indirect communication about the experience of being in trance.

So a client choosing not to dehypnotize may be commenting on the issue that they came to session with ("I'm stuck") OR they may be making a statement about the relationship with you ("I expected having more time with you") OR they may be super suggestible and responding to your very words ("You can come out of hypnosis at a pace that is right for you").

No matter the reason, a sure fire way to bring a person out of the trance is to simply tell them you are going to touch them on the hand only and then wiggle their hand. Alternately, you can reiterate over and over, until the person comes out of trance, the ordinary dehypnotizing suggestions which you will see below.

Here are some examples of typical and everyday ways of bringing a person out of hypnosis:

i.   " You can allow yourself to begin coming out of trance, you can begin cracking your eyes and moving your hands, then opening your eyes wider and moving your arms and moving your legs a little bit, and then you can rise up and wake up all over."

ii.   "You can begin to come up at a very fine pace, perhaps the same way that you get out of bed in the morning when you don't need to hit the snooze alarm, but you don't just jump out. You stretch, open your eyes, and then sit up."

iii.   "You can begin to come out of trance, but do know that when I say come out of trance, what I mean is that you'll be more social, you'll be more physically active, you'll be more mentally active, and more interactive. While all of that happens, you can keep and hold onto all of the good feelings that you have inside, all the relaxation, all the peace of mind, all the feelings of centeredness. Coming out of trance means that you can keep these things in an ongoing way while being more physically mentally and socially active."

If a person does not come out of hypnosis right away you can, as I said earlier, repeat the dehypnotizing instructions a number of times and then tell them you're going to touch their hand and move it and wiggle it while still continuing to suggest that they exit the hypnotic, altered state. Just the same, if you wish to individualize the trance ending instructions, taking into consideration what you deem to be issues you think are central to the situation at hand, then you can say something like what is contained in the two examples below:

i.   "Perhaps you want more time to work with me, and that's why you are remaining in trance. If that is in fact the case, just know that when you come out of hypnosis now we will be making appointments for the future and you're welcome to make as many as you would find useful."

ii. "You want to stay hypnotized. That is just fine. Stay hypnotized for as long as you'd like, 15

Dr. John H. Edgette

minutes or half an hour, even a couple of hours or more. I'm going to see my next patient in the other office so when you do decide to come out of hypnosis simply leave through the waiting room, as you always do."

Now you know how to bring a person out of trance, and in fact know all the stages of hypnosis practice for doing full inductions with volunteers or clients that you are seeing pro bono. After that continue to read about hypnotic phenomena in the chapters to come as they will constitute awesome and most powerful interventions to remediate sexual issues!

PART TWO: GETTING IT ON

CHAPTER 10
Vaginismus Dismissith

The Dildo Song

What rolls downstairs?

Alone or in pairs?

And, makes a buzz-ity sound?

It's long - a schlong - a marvelous dong!

Everyone knows – it's dildo!

What fits in a sock?

Feels better than cock?

And, unlike a man, it's slow

It vibrates a bit

Feels great on your clit

Everyone knows – it's dildo!

"The Dildo Song". A campy, Saturday Night Live type bit. Sung to the tune of "Everyone Knows it's Slinky" See YouTube for the whole song or variations of it.

Vaginismus is a female condition where the opening to the vagina locks or clamps shut in anticipation of penetration. While women often live with this for years or even a lifetime, it is a most curable concern.

The traditional therapeutic approach involves practicing inserting sequentially larger and longer dildo-like probes into the vagina in the hopes that eventually the newfound openness will tide over into and onto the sexual act. Sound like fun? I think not. Quite antiseptic, right?

So why not use real graduated dildos in actual or vividly imagined sexual situations, while immersed in a suitably deep relaxed self-hypnotic state? ***No reason not*** *to!* Besides, it's cheaper. This then is the first hypno-erotic upgrade. For a reminder as to how to perform self- hypnosis, see the earlier chapters on various inductions that can be used. The intervention itself can go something like this: (This induction and intervention needs to be audiotaped because of its nature.)

"As you remain deep in hypnosis you can gently open your eyes a bit while staying in hypnosis and reach over to the first and smallest dildo that you have laid out. As you insert it into yourself, you magically go even deeper into hypnosis. You leave it in there until you feel that you like it in there. You may notice yourself becoming wetter and your juices flowing."

Repeat this type of intervention pattern as the client is instructed to use increasingly larger dildos. When done you can give or send the audiotape to the client. I tape on my iPad with an app that allows me to send the audio file electronically to the consultee.

A second intervention upgrade we can insert entails having the woman in hypnosis imagine (and hence experience) all the hypnotically induced muscle relaxation flowing to her naughty bits. This can be accomplished by having her experience one or multiple water faucets open with warm relaxing water flowing downward from her upper body to her crouch. Alternately, she could envision a rainbow of relaxation steadily forming and bending right toward her "pot of gold". Muscle relaxation is a perfect antidote to a clenched muscle area. It might sound something like this: (Due to the graphic nature of this intervention, it too is best done with audio taping.)

"Water faucets from your shoulders and chest and stomach can open. They can be 3, 4, or even 5 at each level. They can open all at once, simultaneously, or one level at a time. They can be kitchen faucets, bathroom faucets, or an outdoor spigot. They can be ultra-modern in style or very old school. When they open relaxation flows from the various parts of your upper body all the way down to your groin and crotch region. Gently memorize this feeling and lock it in to your permanent memory. By calling up this memory and experiencing it vividly, with all your senses, you can have this experience all over again. Most importantly you can have it whenever you choose to insert something into yourself."

A third fine change strategy involves a woman in self-hypnosis taking herself back in age regression to all the times she inserted something wholly into her honey hole. This commonly might be a tampon or douche. Another ideal experience for her to re-experience anew is that of having a gynecological exam with use of a speculum. This can hold her open, in her imagination as she goes into self-hypnosis and increasingly relaxes around it.

Implementing the third method, delineated above, might sound like this:

"As you go down deeper into hypnosis you can experience yourself going back in time as if you were riding an easily galloping horse through time and you are very relaxed and comfortably astride this animal. Your horse has wings and you fly back in time! From a distance you see down below positive scenes from your life, almost as if they are the only things to view. Then you notice that all the scenes actually entail you inserting something into that sweet and sexy orifice between your legs.

Look! That first tampon, then a parade of tampons thereafter. Light days, heavy days, teen days, scented, unscented, and perhaps once you found a vibrator of a family member, an older sisters or a cousins?

Then maybe a GYN appointment with a trusted doctor. Insertion of this, insertion of that. You may have been nervous at first, probably were, but you learned to relax into it. Who helped you to do that? An aunt, a family friend, your friend, the nurse, the doctor? What did she say and do to put you at ease? You have a long history of comfortable insertion and you can sure remember vividly the feelings associated with those multiple moments and you can bring them back forward to the present and then wonder with curiosity how they will affect the future of insertion."

After this you can reorient a person back to the present by reversing the Pegasus experience delineated. During de-hypnotizing be sure to anchor the person in the present. Alternately, you can proceed with more interventions such as the following:

"And you are deep in hypnosis now. You can enjoy the relaxation in your mind and especially the relaxation in your body. Those muscles of yours are, oh! So relaxed. So you can experience the relaxation in your muscles being of a fluid nature and from your entire upper body that fluid relaxation flows down toward your vagina like tributaries of a stream, of a river, all joining together in one spot. There they coalesce as in a reservoir. They contribute, like a reservoir of relaxation, to an ongoing overall sense of relaxation in that area. Calm, at ease, at peace, a most pleasant feeling. You will be able to hold on to this feeling, in its entirety, through any process of any insertion that you choose to allow."

Here you induce relaxation, move those feelings down to the groin area and give a post hypnotic suggestion to re-experience this when needed. Again, you can choose to end things there or go on with more intervention.

For a novel change intervention, you can **repeat** the exact same script found above. It then becomes a confusion induction (since no one repeats to themselves verbatim, to this extent, in everyday discourse!) as well as a reinforcement of the given suggestions.

CHAPTER 11
Come Again? Male Premature Ejaculation And Female Premature Orgasm

"Relax, don't do it, when you want to go to it........WHEN YOU WANT TO COME." RELAX by Frankie Goes to Hollywood.

Quick cuming can be a problem for some men and a dubious problem for some women. There are cures for both although, for women it really just needs to be managed. Let's address dudes first and save advice for the dudettes for later.

The traditional treatments for men consist of a couple of rather boring and unpleasant activities. The first is called the "squeeze technique". Here the guy or his partner squeezes the top of the dick, just below the head, as the urge to orgasm arises. Repeat as needed. When this works, perhaps it is because it is so unpleasant it takes the fun out of sex, or maybe it works best for masochistic men who like to play "punish the penis".

A second strategy is called the "stop/start technique". Here the man enters the orifice of choice and then withdraws and pauses when he feels the first signs of an orgasm coming on. Repeat as needed, and it is usually needed. It takes discipline. Many give in to the urge to just squirt off. Others don't stop soon enough and spurt their spunk with their eager cock outside their partner. For those who wish to give this method a try it might be useful to first practice while jerking off.

Another traditional and most unsexy cure entails using an anaesthetic cream on the cock to dull sensation. Still yet another strategy is to use a condom or two, whether or not you need to. Yeah right, doesn't everyone love wearing condoms?

One non-hypnotic solution that seems to be working for men and women alike is taking SSRI anti-depressants. These medications are notorious for the sexual side effect of making it difficult to exit the "plateau phase" of arousal and "pull the trigger" in the orgiastic phase. Here it is not a side effect but a side benefit! Talk to your health care provider (by the way, you may want to avoid Viibred because studies and patient reports indicate it might not have the effect mentioned above).

Other non-hypnotic interventions include jerking off every morning or during the lunch hour (this works well and is most fun). After orgasming quickly a man can wait the 45 minutes it takes to recover, on average, and have another go at it. In the meantime, he should be encouraged to not just lay there but to pleasure his partner.

So, what are the hypnotic interventions that can help with cuming too quickly? Well, first there is the use of hypno-anaesthesia. This can be facilitated by using the protocol described in the first portion of this book. This hypnotic phenomena, when pointed toward and consolidated in the prick, will provide a dulling of sensation so that orgasm can be delayed.

Examples of what you might say include, but certainly are not limited to, the following:

"Remember being a child and playing outside in the snow in winter. You have your warm gloves on so your hands get progressively colder and number. Are you building a snowman or an igloo? Having a snowball fight? Anyway, your hands get ever colder and number. You can experience the sensation now, and then you can experience that lack of sensation in your hands, traveling down your arms and your torso into your penis. NOW it would remain for as long as it's useful and just like when you're playing in the snow, you know the numbness will leave later at the appropriate time."

"We all have had the experience of sleeping on our arm and having it "fall asleep", something that you know is safe and will eventually go away given the proper condition. But, until then you can enjoy the novelty of it. Now you can experience that feeling fully. It is familiar and that sensation of numbness can go fully all the way down to your penis right now. It can consolidate and remain there for as long as you like."

For women the situation is quite different. One can even question if there is any such thing as a "premature" orgasm for females. This is because women need only wait, on the average, under a minute, to be ready to orgasm again. So, this fact then invalidates one common definition of this syndrome, that it occurs when a woman comes more quickly then she wishes. She can wait and then come again. Or then again, sometimes a female orgasm is so intense and satisfying that no more are desired.

The other hallmark of this supposed condition is an over sensitivity of the clitoris such that continued sex becomes painful. This, too, is an unnecessary experience because again, the woman can wait a minute or so and then start up again. In the meantime, she should pleasure her partner and not just ignore his or her needs.

Alternately, if she is screwing a guy, or being done with a strap on, she can adopt a sex position where there is little if any clitoral stimulation. It is hard enough for a woman to come while fucking so the right position can make for the avoidance of pain. The position where women get the most stimulation on their button is when they are on top, partially because then they can work the angle so that sensation is maximized. The second most clitoral stimulating position is doggie style. Avoid the above two post orgasm. The missionary position is notoriously devoid of clitoral contact, unless a woman is playing with herself. Thus, picking positions provides potential solutions. Alternately, the couple can do an, uh, end run and switch off and have anal sex after that early orgasm.

If there are still concerns about pain and over sensitivity, the hypno-anesthesia mentioned in the male section above can be utilized. It might sound something like this:

"We all have had the experience of sitting too long in one place and finding that our leg has fallen asleep.

Remember vividly that sensation now and amazingly you can find it is all traveling up your leg and consolidating in your clit, making it numb until you decide to call off that loss of sensation."

Alternately, the non-hypnotic solutions discussed for men can be utilized by women as well. Here, I am referring of course to stop/start, numbing creams (keep it away from the guys cock unless you both come faster than you like!), SSRI's, and morning masturbation. Stay away from the squeeze method, for obvious reasons!

CHAPTER 12
Navigating Erectile Dysfunction Junction

"Anyone who thinks 'all men are created equal' has never been to a nude beach." Dr. John H. Edgette.

Even in this era of Viagra and related drugs, men crave harder and longer lasting erections, some men just want to have one (yes, you can even remain flaccid with vitamin V) and while there are a number of prostheses available, they are expensive and often awkward to use. Moreover, using an external device, such as a vacuum pump, is as unsexy as having sex wearing a c-pap machine (that being said I'm betting there is, or soon will be, a website called C-Papsex.com). Furthermore, cock rings can be dangerous to use.

An excellent way to help your client is to use hypnosis and is most effective. First off, in hypnosis and out, I always avoid using the term "erectile dysfunction" because it is gratuitously pseudo-scientific. Instead I use the phrase "getting a better and longer lasting erection" because it is professional while not being sterile. Note: I don't say "getting an erection" because it promotes all or nothing thinking which is counterproductive to solution focused success. The phrase I use allows for incremental progress and hence a therapeutic focus on process and not outcome.

Once hypnosis begins, I like using the phrase "going deeper" because it has a duel meaning: going deeper into trance and an erection going deeper during sex. Also, during hypnosis, I don't hesitate to use slang terms like "boner", "woodie", and "hard on" because I have already established myself as a professional consultant during the initial interview by using the word "erection".

I do, however, let the client know in advance that I will be using guttural words. The benefit of using slang is that it more easily allows for change because it is sensory and not cerebral. It is far easier to accomplish the mission at hand by accepting into the subconscious "hardening, engorging, and elongating the one-eyed snake" then it is by saying "your phallus can get erect". Yet prudes will balk, but prudes will loosen up therapeutically via this method.

Here is a protocol for accomplishing the above. First, hypnotize your subject using an induction you think they will respond to. If the client is slow to go into trance, then use multiple inductions (see chapter x).

Then you can ratify their trance state as a positive reinforcement and to deepen the hypnosis (see chapter x).

After that you may educate the client regarding the optimal mind set with which to accept the hypnotic suggestions (see chapter x).

Following that you can begin to give suggestion for change. You can pick any combination of the following or develop your own.

One of my favorites is to increase blood flow to the organ in question. In hypnosis blood flow can be regulated to an amazing extent. During surgery people can make it such that less blood is lost. Phantom limb pain can be relieved by moving blood to the site of the amputation. Breasts can be enlarged. Circulation problems, including Renaud's disease, can be relieved. I have personally enabled a phlebotomist to find a vein to draw blood from when I was dehydrated and it was difficult to find. After the vein was discovered, it made the blood draw easier and faster. Hence, engorging an organ should be a lay-up; this includes the female naughty bits as well because it makes for more powerful female orgasms.

Start more blood flow to the male member by first having the client experience a warmth down below, as if it were being warmed by a fire from afar. Perhaps a campfire or a fireplace. Suggest the warmth increas over time.

Blood flow can also be increased to create a stiffy by imagining a water faucet at the base of the dick. This can be a modern faucet, a classic one, or both. Alternately, a garden hose can be experienced emanating from the torso while getting ever more rigid.

As you may notice from the above change strategies it is good to use as many synonyms for erections as possible. This facilitates the desired result by directly suggesting an erection in multiple ways, imbedded in the broader intervention.

It is also a good idea to emphasize **effortlessness** throughout. This quality is essential to optimal sexual functioning, woody development included. This can be done by using words such as "easy" or "casual" or "laid back" or implied in a metaphor. For example, experience this metaphor which is an adaptation and elaboration of one told by Milton Erickson: " It is so very easy to become deeply relaxed while gardening, the outside world can just fade away. You prepare fertile soil, it's important that it be moist. You ensure optimal lighting and when the time is right plant the seed deep, and you do this repeatedly, thrusting over and over, in the bed and over time you tend to this garden, you do it regularly so there is no rush."

"AND NO ONE EVER GREW A PROPER PLANT BY PULLING AND TUGGING ON THE STEM TO MAKE IT GROW......."

Although it shouldn't need to be said, I'll say it anyway, relaxation is the most important thing to repeatedly emphasize during the hypnotic treatment of someone with difficulty getting an erection. Although hypnosis without any goal at all will naturally, and by definition, include relaxation, one should emphasize it throughout and deepen the experience. Bluntly stated, relaxation makes any shaft harder and longer lasting!

"Sensate Focus" should also be a cornerstone of any seduction of a better boner. This technique, first developed by Masters and Johnson, is quite simple. It entails the helpful partner serially and increasingly teasing the male so as to elicit the, sometimes, elusive erection. Every night, or every couple of nights, the couple does a bit more sexually, only touching the dick at the very end of the protocol. No orgasm is allowed until the very, very, end either.

Masturbation should not take place for days prior to the start of the above protocol. The couple starts off with a half hour kissing session and this progresses over the days to increasing amounts of body touching, never including direct touching of the male meat. Erections will happen, yet nothing is done about it! Sex is avoided, not only during, but after the sessions as well. Eventually though, the functioning erection is put into an orifice, but no movement should take place. Orgasm may occur, and that is fine, no worries about future premature ejaculation. In following sessions movement can occur and the remedy should be complete. However, should difficulty obtaining a steely occur, couples can go back to the first step and repeat the procedure more slowly.

Also know that sometimes couples "disobey Dr's orders" and can't resist having sex early on in the therapeutic sequence. That is to be expected! When the consultant learns this, he or she should encourage the couple NOT to give in to the temptation to complete the sex act. This soft prohibition can however actually prove therapeutic. Partners often revel that in "disobeying" the authority the erections thereby became more robust and the "sneaky" fucking was more fun.

Note that sensate focus entails an element of therapeutic paradox. This is because the very idea that you cannot culminate the sex act makes it hard to NOT get hard!

You can actually paradox your client in more direct and standard ways. For example, you can give him the homework assignment to TRY not to GET HARD. Note that here the word "try" is therapeutic by carrying the usual connotation that the effort will be unsuccessful. Attend also to the imbedded message "get hard" which contains the admonition to fail at the task of staying soft.

Needless to say, all of the above, including sensate focus, can be suggested and prescribed within a hypnotic session. In fact, that is what makes this work more powerful than using those interventions solo. It is important to know that there is a subtype of ED that requires special and different interventions. This subtype entails the LOSS of the erection AFTER obtaining it and often during sex proper (or should I say improper?).

This happens because the valves that keep the blood in the phallus leak. Yup, whereas younger men have seals that hold in the blood that has flowed to the erect dick and engorged it, older men can have "worn out" and looser seals that fail at this task.

Yet there are actually numerous physiological reasons why this syndrome may occur. Venous leak can be caused by OR and is linked to many conditions, most often vascular disease, which is most commonly caused by diabetes. Venous leak is also linked to scar tissue, nerve issues, and even anxiety. If you suspect any of these conditions are the cause of the issue it is best that you consult with an urologist. Just the same, having any of these conditions does not preclude hypnotic treatment. It is just that there may be other compatible medical remedies to help the client. Also, hypnosis can be individualized to any diagnosed physical condition other than ageing (e.g. giving suggestions for weight loss, dietary changes, and increased exercise for the diabetic).

A non-psychological intervention that can be useful for venous leak is the use of a "cock ring". It will be easier for the reader to Google a picture of this device than to have me describe it. Because it is actually two connected rings at different angles such that one supports the balls from behind and the other the base of the ever stiffening or already stiff member.

A purchased cock ring should be either snap off or sufficiently stretchy such that it can never do its job too well and be difficult to take off. Rings that remain on too long can cause permanent damage to the dong. Opinions vary as to how long is too long, so obviously great care should be taken to ensure it is removed well before the most conservative deadline. Hospital emergency rooms and paramedics worldwide have become all too accustomed to cutting these off, often with special devices!

One legendary hypnosis colleague of mine once stated, "The worst thing that can happen during hypnosis is that nothing happens." Since that is the case, clearly hypnotic interventions should be used prior to the deployment of this devise.

The most effective line of intervention for leaky valve syndrome is to employ select metaphors to alleviate the problem at hand. One that I have successfully utilized includes the idea of an air mattress being blown up after having been patched to fix a leak. Images of properly patched tire tubes and above ground pools are very helpful as well. If the person is knowledgeable about cars the hypnotist can speak about car gaskets being fixed, or leaky oil, brake, or steering wheel fluid seals being remediated. Likewise, if someone is into home improvements then you can speak in terms of fixing a leak in the roof or basement, or caulking a water seeping bathtub.

Whether by metaphor or therapeutic task assignment or both, erectile dysfunction, physical or psychological, can be successfully treated with hypnosis.

CHAPTER 13
Male and Female Delayed Orgasm Treated Hypnotically "Can We Get This Over With Anytime Soon?"

"Sometimes I wonder if men and women really suit each other. Perhaps they should live next door and just visit now and then." Actress Katherine Hepburn

A client once complained that his wife hated how long it would take him to cum. After what seemed to be an endless period of time (it probably wasn't really that long since the AVERAGE length of time till ejaculation is two minutes!). She would rather dryly suggest that he "get it over with" so she could go do something else. Rather difficult to cum under those circumstances, no? Well, she finally got wise and emotionally generous in saying "go ahead and close your eyes and pretend you are fucking Susie." He would then come almost immediately!

My client was on an anti-depressant that is an SSRI, which is an abbreviation for "selective serotonin reuptake inhibitor". For both males and females, this category of medication is notorious for making it difficult to climax. Both sexes complain about how hard it is to "pull the trigger". They get stuck in what is called the plateau phase of the sexual act.

My client's partner, mentioned above, inadvertently stumbled upon one of the best ways to "overcome" delayed ejaculation. This method works just dandy to help women cum or to cum more easily as well. It entails deep, sensory absorption in an erotic fantasy. In the example above the partner knew of my client's attraction to "sexy Susie", as they called her. So sexy Susie was invoked such that she became Susie Surrogate!

Fantasy is best when shared and enhanced by the banter or enactment of one's partner. It can be kept private though if the nature of it would prove problematic to one's mate. Either way, it is important to strongly emphasize to oneself or as a dyad that there is an essential, very critical, and most needed distinction between what one fantasizes about and what one actually does in real life. If the client/clients can't do that for themselves then this notion should be introduced and buttressed by you, the hypnotic consultant. Words and ideas matter, and here they can matter even more if embedded in the hypnotic experience. Thus, hypnosis can help a person have fantasies, vivify their fantasies, make them more creative, and obviate unneeded guilt. Guilt can unnecessarily attenuate or eliminate erotic pleasure and hence orgiastic ecstasy. But again, while some people will need encouragement to ever more boldly enact what they desire, many will need to leave it be as a fantasy. NOT EVERYONE SHOULD LIVE

OUT THIER LEWD SEX SCENARIOS! And when in doubt it's best to shrug it off.

Absorption in fantasy means leaving the reality of the connection to your partner. While this relational psychological commitment is ideal for close and intimate every day and every night interactions, it is antithetical to hot kinky sex. Getting to know ever more deeply the same daily other is increasingly satisfying for an existential, enduring, and spiritual love. Yet that very detailed and differentiated knowledge that actualizes the truest love, makes sex incredibly boring. We grow weary, tired, and unexcited by routine and repetition of personhood. We become enlivened and turned-on by difference, newness, the unexpected, and unconquered uniqueness. Good sex and good love are utterly different experiences and are accomplished via two very different pathways.

I'll recount an interaction that took place at a seminar where I was to discuss sexuality with another leading figure in the field. It became something of a debate in actuality. When the other presenter said something to the effect that "one of the best ways to enhance orgasm is to look deeply into your partners eyes as you experience release." My response? "The only time a person should have their eyes open during sex is when they are cuming while driving and getting road head or road finger." The audience of mostly staid professionals gasped.

Here are examples of what can be said in hypnosis to foster a fantastic release via fantasy:

"As you go down deeper and deeper into hypnosis your unconscious mind will automatically unleash formidable erotic experiences that turn you on tremendously. They will bubble up like carbonation rising up in seltzer as the cap is slowly removed. Some of you will recognize this from when you get yourself off, while others may be new and provide luscious possibilities for exploration using all your senses. What is the smell like? Is there a unique and particular taste? Oh the touch, the feel! The view!"

"You told me you are curious about BDSM. You have had some experience you say. Absorb yourself in the special smell of leather, what it is like to run your hand over quality leather, see the beauty of a finally crafted flogger that is mainly black with subtle yet present red piping, the sound of a proper spanking, the sound of the single tail cracking, the feel of the back and forth motion of the flogger. Think of these things in full sensory bloom as you decide to allow yourself to give in to orgiastic release."

Besides fantasy, the other great way to help clients come more quickly is to increase the sensitivity of the organs of orgasm. This holds true for both men and woman. It is very achievable by thought and intention alone for a very imaginative and suggestible person. But easier, still, is to make it a reality via hypnosis using hyperesthesia. This is the opposite of anaesthesia and entails enhanced tactile sensing. More about this hypnotic phenomena and how to elicit it can be found by revisiting the earlier chapters of this book. For now though, savor these sample suggestions as to how to increase the sensations that will co-create climax.

"Just as everyone has had times when their skin has been duller or even numb, they also have had times when they have been more exquisitely sensitive to touch. Less sensitive when you have a callous, a blister, or a part of your body that is worn and toughened up. More sensitive when you gently focus on the body part that touches something else and you purposefully turn up the magic dial that will increase the sensation. This dial can go from 1 to 10 and have a little notch below each number on the dial. Move it up to number three or four and see the exquisite increase in tactile feeling."

"In the Far East there are certain people that, for curious reasons, believe that less stimulation to the genitalia is somehow desirable for spiritual development. They wear something akin to a diaper with a gaping area in front that precludes tactile contact with clothes. On the other hand, here in the west, there are men and women who wear underwear that purposefully stimulates the clit or cock by contact. By wearing such garments you can experience that effect and I would like you to, here in hypnosis, recognize that your vivid memory or imagination can create or recreate those very sensations in the here and the now."

"Men and woman alike do various things to their naughty bits to invite them to be more sensually alive. Gay men pioneered the notion of shaving their balls to increase stimulation and one has to wonder if the required focus of attention on their nut sack also serves to enhance sensation as well. Women will put ben wa balls of various sizes and textures into their southernmost orifice to stimulate themselves throughout a day to give an erotic surge to an otherwise mundane schedule. Likewise, women will sometimes get the hood of their clit pierced with a horizontal rod with a small rolling stainless steel ball riding in the middle. Clitoral stimulation makes for an easier cum, whether via actuality or imaginarily (sic) these sensations and stimulations can be reliably realized, and you will discover just how much simulation becomes realization (sic)."

"And we haven't even begun to discuss panty vibrators, remote or wired. We haven't even started to imagine (sic) all the varieties of butt plugs that guys and gals will employ and deploy to explode with exotic erotic glee and the vast array of nipple piercings and nipple clips that both sexes will use to urge on libidinal and volcanic like sexual energy."

So, for you, the reader, to support the learnings elucidated above it would be useful for you to take time and create your own hypnotic scripts that, of course, have the potential to be individualized to the client at hand. Remember, of course, that in this chapter we are focusing on the twin interventions of creating and enhancing fantasy and also stimulation all in service of fostering faster finales.

CHAPTER 14
Diagnose Or They Will Quickly Say Adios: Refined Hypnosis For Delayed Orgasm

"Having sex with a new partner is a diagnostic endeavor. To have it be good you root around for what they like and don't like. You see what turns them on and what makes them stiffen. It is an adventure of diagnosing the ways an individual experiences pleasure. In contrast, in mental health you are diagnosing the ways a person creates their own misery." Dr. John Edgette

Dr. John H. Edgette

A reader who had heard of my work e-mailed me with a question that illustrates the need for an accurate understanding of the underlying cause of a disorder. While, many times, a sexual issue can be resolved in a simple and straightforward way, at other times a unique and particular mechanism underlies the difficulty. So, how to know? How to proceed?

In the initial discussion and interview about the sexual complaint the special considerations may become apparent. This is what happens in the three example paragraphs below.

At other times trying the most obvious change strategy first is the best way to proceed. Then, if the problem does not resolve, think about addressing an alternative cause for it. Years ago many successful corporations switched from a "ready, aim, fire" model to a "ready, fire, aim" approach. That is what you are doing with this second approach to cure.

In any event, here is the e-mail and the response. An initial understanding of the problem is followed by a game plan for a hypnotic solution.

Cindy: I am e-mailing you about a friend of mine who has been dating a man who is a widower. He gets an erection but is having difficulty having an orgasm with her (his girlfriend) because he keeps on thinking about his late wife.

Any solutions for them?

I appreciate your input! Thanks in advance.

Dr. John: Thanks for writing. Most happy to help. You pretty much have handed me the diagnosis of the problem. Yet there are some rule-outs that need to be considered because they could cause or exacerbate the issue at hand. After the death of his wife, did he go on an SSRI antidepressant? The sexual side-effects could be contributing to his difficulty. Secondly, per-chance did his wife die during the sex act? I assume not but if it were so, the therapy would be simple, targeted, but intense. It would best involve deep hypnosis to separate the experience of death from the experience of sex via a robust and unbreachable dissociation. Lastly, in a more general way, is there additional grief work that needs to be done? If so, it can be done, without a focus on sex, if the following simpler change strategies do not work. But as a matter of fact, the solution strategy described below may actually indirectly foster any needed mourning.

With the above considerations in mind there is a plan A and then a backup plan B. I will elucidate, the next time I e-mail you.

C: He doesn't take any meds.

His wife died of cancer in a hospital, so I doubt it was during the act. I'm not certain about the grief work. She died about 15 months ago. He tells my friend that she was the "love of my life". So very sweet and he has gone to a therapist and talks about his dead wife frequently. My friend tells me he frequently says it was one of the hardest things he's ever done: watching and taking care of his dying wife.

J: That is very sweet and tender. Unfortunately, that sentiment is probably the very thing that is holding him back. It is almost as if he is telling your friend so to give her a heads up as to what is to come, or not come, in this case.

First off, I would suggest to your friend that she should encourage him to cultivate the mental discipline not to think of his deceased wife during sex. This is a decision he should gently but clearly suggest to himself in a contemplative moment prior to sex. Then he should have sex in a **VERY** different fashion from how he did with his deceased wife. Different places, positions, acts, and fantasies, etc. He would be well advised to gently, but with intentionality, focus on the UNIQUE and distinct aspects of his new partners sensory personhood. How her hair smells, the scent of her body, the color and texture of her hair (everywhere she has hair), the detailed differences of her sex-body; how her breasts, clit, and other sex-bits are special and individualized to her and her alone. The distinct taste, smell, texture, wetness, and swelling of her welcoming orifice and all the while how his current partner has nipples that are utterly unique to her, as unique as a fingerprint or snowflake.

Ok, anyway, you get the idea. During sex there should be a full and gentle yet persistent sensory focus on this new woman in his life. The central idea is to sever the associations between his beloved deceased wife and the sex act. All the while honouring her memory while accepting the invitation for his future of alternate love.

C: Thank you so much. I think this will be helpful to her.

J: U are most welcome.

Plan B would be the backup and a bit more radical but most effective if it needs to be employed. It is somewhat the opposite of the above. It entails him envisioning, vividly, again in a contemplative moment, his beloved deceased wife giving him permission to enjoy sex with his new partner. I'm even guessing that this is what she would want for him anyway. And after all, most of us do, from time to time, in the heat of masturbation or sex, think of the heat we once had with others who have passed on or have simply moved on. All of the above requires clear communication, comprehension, and trust. After all it is going from me to you to her to him. So, if for any reason it does not translate properly thru the chain into change, he is most welcome to take a sexology consult with me via phone, FaceTime, or Zoom. This would have the added benefit of allowing the introduction of hypnosis as a most potent turbocharger for change. Again, I am very happy to offer my help here.

Oh yes, if after utilizing the above change strategies this issue has not resolved there may be a need for even more information gathering. For example, it may be relevant to know if he has trouble cuming while masturbating. If not, what is it that he allows himself to think about or experience or not experience that allows him to cum?

C: I think this is a super advice doctor. I am confident it will help. I can't thank you enough.

The above is just one example of how to discern the exact intervention to employ. You can start with the obvious and go from there unless you have important information that leads you in a different direction. But if you start with the obvious and get nowhere it is best to dig for particularities that you need to know in order to cure. Here plan A entailed creating a therapeutic dissociation leading to orgasm while plan B involved fostering an association leading to release.

103

It is essential to note that the above thinking has been applied to delayed orgasm as a complaint. THE WAY OF THINKING DEPLOYED APPLIES TO WORK WITH ALL ISSUES AND PROBLEMS, SEXUAL AND OTHERWISE! Moreover, it is also relevant to resolving barriers people face related to cutting loose and experiencing ever new sexual heights and freedoms, the hypnotic exotic that is erotic.

In summary, diagnose or your client will soon say adios!!!

CHAPTER 15
Very Delayed Female Orgasm: Anorgasmia

"Really that little deal bob is too far away from the hole. It should be built right in."

Country singer Loretta Lynn (not afraid to get literal about the clitoral).

The term "anorgasmia" is rather rotten, no? Not only does it refer to the problem and not the event-to-be but it also pathologies a simple mind - body disconnect that can be easily remediated. Plus, the absurdity of the very word (like the use of Latin terms to describe basic phobias) seems designed to allow slews of professionals to feel really scientific when using it. I prefer the term "pre orgasmic". Note that this term contains a presupposition that the woman will in fact eventually cum.

Whatever you call it, this issue can be defined as a woman's seeming inability to have an orgasm, given proper stimulation. More on the stimulation issue in a moment.

It is interesting that there are no case reports of this problem in men. Men can actually ejaculate and orgasm without getting an erection. Perhaps, the issue of ED is so primary that orgasmic capability is overlooked if not overcome.

Above there was a reference to "easily remediated". Yup, it is true. Especially when certain personal and sociocultural taboos and inhibitions are put aside. The most common cause of delayed orgasm is insufficient foreplay. Women are vastly different from men in this regard. They need much more foreplay to get within range of cumming. In fact, studies have repeatedly shown that gay women (and men) have a much greater level of sexual satisfaction then hetero couples because they engage in far more foreplay.

Milton Erickson, the father of modern clinical hypnosis, often encouraged couples in this fashion. An ultra-conservative couple came to him because of dissatisfaction with their sex life. Erickson discerned that the reason was that they were just rushing into screwing. They needed more foreplay. Because they were prudish, he deemed it unwise to address the issue directly. Instead, he used the indirect method of metaphor for the intervention, utilising their love of another activity that gets the mucous membrane activity pumping. In what follows, note that embedded suggestions are italicised. Paraphrasing, Erickson said "You prefer to go to *fine* restaurants and you don't just sit down and order up the first thing you see. You generally *wait* to be seated, and while you do you might gaze at a sample menu, ***allowing the anticipation to grow***. When you do sit, you still don't order right off and dive right in, but instead you allow the wait to make the eventual meal all that more satisfying. You do however order up a cocktail, **taking your time,** allowing those salivary **juices to begin flowing** more and more. You listen to the specials and fantasize as to what you might enjoy devouring but you don't just order two entries and dig right in. Instead, you order a couple of appetisers and continue the **adventure in consumption** and all the while **all your senses come alive**. The **smells** from the chef **cooking** in the kitchen delights, **things are really heating up now**. The texture on your tongue is **luscious** as you **share** your **warm-up dish**, back and forth, **alternating reciprocally**." You get the idea, I am sure! He actually would go on and on seemingly endlessly (he could really last), through desert and the after dinner drink and even the talking on the long ride home. Follow-up with the couple years later showed that the intervention was highly successful.

A second strategy for resolving preorgasmia has to do with female fantasizing. While most men are comfortable with erotic fantasies, women sometimes have been taught that it is wrong or "sinful" to think "impure thoughts". Yet they are natural, fun, and healthy, and can bring forth one's best and most creative sexual self. See chapter __ for ways to help a client rid themselves of unwanted guilt, shame, and inhibitions. It is important to reiterate here that there can be a hugantic differences between what one fantasizes about and what one actually does. Elsewhere we will talk about how to know the difference and how to test out whether to act on a fantasy. It varies year to year in surveys, but typically the most popular female fantasies involve anonymous sex, gang bangs, and even rape. While role playing with a trusted partner or partners, only a few would actually want to enact the first two scenarios and none the last. Yet shame and guilt should not delimit the sexual pleasure that can be had once a person understands that thoughts and actions are different and will only intermingle upon sober, sensible, and conscious vetting, and after finding ways to test the waters first. More on all this, elsewhere.

Fantasies can be discovered, enriched, and elaborated quite easily in hypnosis. This will allow them to surface (for the person who is having difficulty accessing them) or to be enlivened (for those who have them but want a more vivid and differentiated experience). For an example: how hypnosis can turbocharge imaginable sexuality see chapter __ which consists of a transcript of a group induction designed to unleash sexual desire and adventurousness as well as fantasy.

Male and females tend to employ different ways of fantasizing. Men tend to be visual and like to watch videos and look at pictures. Women tend to like to read erotica or more commonly use ideation or visual imagery to get turned on and/or get off. Yet these tendencies seem to be shifting as role and gender stereotypes shift. For example, Good Vibrations (goodvibes.com) is a sex positive, women owned and operated sexuality store. In addition to sex toys and collections of written erotica, they have sex positive, women respectful movies. Titles such as "Back Door Boyfriend" bemuse some (about a girl with a strap on and her guy who enjoys "pegging") as do "40 Years Old, Comes to Life" and "Interracial Transsexuals - Part 2".

Speaking of Good Vibrations, they are a leading online purveyor of the items that constitute the third way for a woman to create a cme:; sex toys! Combined with fantasy, it is very much the time for a total blast off, or two, or three, or more. Go to goodvibes.com (and no, there is no sponsorship from them for this book) and see the vast array of dildos and vibrators that are available for purchase. Big and small, battery or electric, remote or manual, the choices are endless. Something for every woman! Want waterproof? It's there! Want one that is embedded in a panty and can be controlled wirelessly from afar by another? Clients are but a credit card away from it being delivered overnight! The result? Artesian orgasms! Nervous, first time buyers can relax about delivery to their door, sex toys come to you in a plain brown wrapper with the return address unremarkable.

Only a rare few women can cum without any clitoral stimulation. Some can cum by manual or oral means given by another. Many can orgasm via using their own fingers. Easiest though is to use a vibrator. Why not? Technology exists to make life easier and orgasms easier too! And don't say that you don't need one, implying that all you need is a dick (or dick head). This isn't a dick verses vibrator competition. Anyway of cuming is a good way! Anytime is a good time for any type of orgasm! And do get the guys to relax - only the most insecure or inept would believe that the buzz tool will replace them.

One last consideration: Position. Very few women can orgasm while screwing. The ones that can do so most easily while on top or doing it doggy style. This is because of enhanced clitoral stimulation in these positions. On top, a woman can adjust her angle to make the grind just as she likes it. When getting it from behind the "hood", over the clit slides back and forth creating very pleasurable sensations, sometimes leading to orgasm. The missionary position, (invented by guess whom?) is far and away the all-time worst in terms of eliciting female orgiastic potential. Yet even while using "best practices" sex positions orgasming is easier when there is finger stimulation from oneself or one's partner. Fingering yourself or being fingered while screwing often can make the big "O" happen or happen more easily. Fingering oneself can result in "Organic Orgasms"!

A woman can also easily use vibrators to touch herself while using these positions! Easily you say? Yup! Our friends at Good Vibrations offer at least one type of mini vibrator that is like a latex mini glove that goes over the middle finger and does its job unobtrusively. So, you need not worry about dick to pussy interference from humongous sized super powerful vibrators.

Ok, to summarise, you lay the groundwork with your consultee, encouraging them to use hypnotically enhanced foreplay and fantasy activity. Then, during a masturbatory moment, she could deploy those dirty thoughts, while employing her superb sex toy. While fucking, she could do all of the above while using pOwer pOsitions.

Notice how we have gone from having your client have a first time orgasm to entertaining the wondrous notion of how many, how powerful, and in which way? We presuppose success and so it will be!

CHAPTER 16
Deconstructing Unwanted Guilt, Shame and Inhibitions: Hypnotic Suggestions for Remodeling Your Conscience

"Dedicated to the countless men and women who have fought the lonely battle against guilt for doing sex acts that are neither harmful to themselves or others." Albert Ellis, Sex without Guilt.

In writing that dedication to his 1958 landmark book, Albert Ellis stepped up as one of the earliest mental health practitioners to sound a rallying cry for the active removal of unneeded sexual restraint. While most often thought of as one of the founding fathers of cognitive behavior therapy, this classic book identifies him as part of the triumvirate, with Kinsey and Hefner, that kick started the sexual revolution.

Albert Ellis saved my sexual life. To this day, this remains my idea as to how to best be "saved"! As an utterly inhibited and guilt ridden 16 year old Catholic boy with an interest in psychology, I somehow stumbled across this book. Without the aid of hypnosis and being horridly un-suggestible to boot, my motivation, need, and determination enabled me nonetheless to kneed the healing messages into my sex-soul.

Hypnosis, however, does make this task much smoother, easier, and more doable. It is the tool that allows what a person's conscious-mind-best-self deems needed to become operational at a subconscious and visceral level.

Many rather intimidating tones have been written about the origins and vicissitudes of guilt and inhibitions. All are not useful and even iatrogenic in a sense though because an in depth knowledge of a problematic attitude will only afford us opportunity to eloquently create more of the same. In a healing solution focused life, attention needs to be paid primarily to deconstructing and removing inhibitions. Simply put, what we need to know about guilt and inhibitions is that they are often generated by well-intentioned parents, clergy, medical professionals, and the like who use their power, authority, and influence to encourage individuals feel badly about harmless erotic desires. Frequently young and/or vulnerable, these messages are often received while the person is in a very impressionable and even hypnotic like state. Childhood and church have often combined to create corrosive constraints. Enter hypnosis- the ultimate process to allow for a demolition of these limitations, and then a construction of a desired erotic self.

Shame is similar to guilt in often unnecessarily limiting orgiastic pleasure. While guilt involves a person's internalized conscience berating of oneself for actions performed or wishes entertained, shame is the feeling that arises as one considers the real or imagined judgments of others vis-á-vis these same desires or behaviors. Shame often needlessly limits or blocks full sexual pleasure.

Guilt and shame are not always undesirable experiences however. Guilt and shame, when needed but absent, allow perpetrators to take advantage of drunk women and men, adulating altar boys and girls, and idealizing graduate students as well as many others. Shame and guilt should only be obliterated when then a person can have safe, sane, and consensual sex-fun. Importantly, guilt and shame also can be invaluable in allowing one to be true to thought out, examined, and desired values endorsed by an adult's conscious mind and best self. Moreover, it can serve one in helping preclude involvement in wild and wooly erotic situations that a person is not emotionally ready to handle at present or perhaps ever. For example, someone who is characteristically insecure, jealous, and possessive is best off eschewing the temptation to watch their spouse being pleasured by another. When self-awareness and good judgment fail, guilt and shame can be a fine friend!

Apart from these cautionary points though, it is now time to proclaim: "LET THE GAMES BEGIN!"

But just how you ask? Well, the very first step is to shed one's unneeded and unwanted shame and guilt baggage. Enter the very powerful tool of hypnosis in service of re-deciding what values you wish to allow to control your erotic adventures. At last you control this psychic event, not the bishop when you were 8, the teacher when you were 12, the parents when you were 14, or the gynecologist when you were 18.

- Here then is the protocol to follow to effect changes that will obviate burdensome guilt and shame.
- First, as always, do a hypnotic induction (Chapters 2,3,4,5).
- Second, adopt an openness to suggestion (Chapter 7).

Third, develop metaphors and hypnotic phenomena to destroy old and delimiting sexual dictates (Chapter 8).

The first two procedures you already know how to perform. Below find script examples of how to create the third step.

"You can allow yourself to experience in front of you a fire into which you throw the contents of your unwanted inhibitions. They can appear in contract form and be torn apart by you prior to tossing the bits into the flames."

"You can experience yourself holding a contract that contains sexual prohibitions that you no longer find relevant or useful. You dig a ditch in a field and, after ripping up the contract, you bury it there. You then erect a small marker which records the approximate dates the prohibitions were put on you along with today's date. Above that you write or sculpt, 'Rest in Peace'. You can then go whole and write up a new contract that nullifies the first contract and sets forth the sexual principles you now wish to live by."

"You can go back in time until you are once again with the individual who is giving you messages that are guilt inducing regarding sex. You shake your head NO and tell him or her that they are misguided and they themselves have problems and hang-ups. You then tell them you are not going to follow their advice"

Suggestions like these deconstruct and thereby destroy old and unhelpful dictates that inhibit a healthy sexuality. Therefore, they serve as ideal preludes to suggestions for a free and unencumbered sexual self. These come aplenty in the chapter that follows.

CHAPTER 17
Robust Sexual Desire: A Robust Live Transcript

"My mother said it was simple to keep a man; you must be a maid in the living room, a cook in the kitchen, and a whore in the bedroom. I said I'd hire the first two and take care of the bedroom bit." Jerry Hall, sharing her strategy for encouraging mate Mick Jagger to spend some quality time at home.

Below the reader will find a full transcript containing embedded or subliminal suggestions designed to promote a fuller sexuality and thereby an increase and robust sexual desire. It was given as a group induction to a large gathering of trainees in hypnosis. The interspersed and embedded suggestions are noted by bold type. As an exercise in hypnotic self-improvement see if you can find some subliminal suggestions that were overlooked by the author and therefore were not in bold type.

The group induction begins:

"Hypnosis is a way in which *you can get beyond the constraints that bind you*. So that is what we are going to be doing today. Some ground rules are as follows. I have the expectation that all of you will do your best to take care of yourselves. If in hypnosis, I say something that you don't feel comfortable with, you are free to ignore it or certainly modify it or change it so that it is suitable to you. Unlike an individual induction, I can't tailor things to each of you in the room. We are having a group experience here. As is the case with any group experience, the individual participant needs to monitor what is going on for them and adjust it accordingly.

I'd like people to **remain open** and remember that during hypnosis anything that occurs or happens to you in fantasy is something that you can be open to. Fantasy is something worth exploring so that you can take a look at and use it as a vehicle for understanding yourself. A vehicle for self-development via hypnosis.

What I'd like you to consider doing is going into trance today in a way that is different for you. **Doing it in a different fashion than you've been doing it.** You've been here for a couple of days and have had a lot of experiences and most of you have had a significant amount of experience previously. If not, most of you are at least journeymen and journeywomen. I think that hypnosis, like sex, is something that can become routine and stagnant. You can wind up doing the same inductions over and over again. One of the ways I circumvent is that I encourage my students and supervisors is to **do something different each time**, each week that they are doing hypnosis.

You are certainly welcome to do this with your eyes open if that is what you'd like to do, if that is novel for you. You can focus some spot on the wall, on the floor, your hands or something you choose. Mrs. Erickson used to go into hypnosis by focusing on her diamond engagement ring. She would focus on it, then defocus on it with her eyes, and then begin to head down into trance. If you haven't done it with your eyes open, I would certainly encourage it. It would keep you somewhat more reality bound at first. Sometimes it's easier and more pleasant. But for others you find it easier to relax when your eyes are closed and allow whatever will bubble up to bubble up. But again, I will leave that up to you. I think that it is a good idea to do hypnosis in a different way so that it doesn't become the same old, same old, boring thing. It's a good idea to avoid hypnotic burn out the same way it's important to avoid sexual burn out.

As you begin to **go down** and as you begin to notice certain feelings of relaxation to come over you, you can also allow yourself to focus on the sound of my voice. Remember, as I said before, you are also free to modify that. The hypnotic experience is a co-constructed experience. I contribute some things and I'll try to say and do things that are conducive to a positive experience on your part. You can allow yourself to hear other hypnotic voices that were supportive and that engender a fuller trance response on your part in your person hood. So, those experiences from your past that you might want to utilize, this can be, this might be, this should be a group induction that involves more than one hypnotist so you can hear voices of other people that have hypnotized you. You can even add your own hypnotic voice to this experience and how is it that you can think back and reflect back on other times when you enjoyed the hypnotic experience the most. What was it about that experience that was so satisfying, so pleasurable?

You can meander in this and think to yourself, what happened then that was particularly good for me? Was it the way in which the person was leading the hypnosis? It is *usually someone that leads or initiates.* Even in self-hypnosis there is a part of you that decides where to go and what to do, and it's good to have intention and not be casual about it. It's also good to be *open and creative* about it.

Dr. John H. Edgette

Listen to your subconscious mind. It's one of the advantages of hypnosis that when it comes to opening up and freeing up our sexuality, it puts us in touch with a very creative part of ourselves. There are certainly other parts of ourselves that can observe with interest and fascination. Especially in regard with what it is that we want to experience or that we have yet to experience.

There are many hypnotic phenomena that so many people don't allow themselves to sample. Hypnosis and sexuality can be like going into a Baskin Robbins and taking one of those tiny sampler spoons and trying a flavor that you haven't yet tried. How do you ever know if you'd like Double Fudge Peanut Brittle Vanilla Chunk if you have never as much as taken a little sample of it? *You can feel free to sample and try on for size different things in your mind.* Fantasy is not the same as reality and any one fantasy may not be the one you'd want to try out. Certainly living life hypnotically might not be the best thing. Walking around hypnotized 24/7 in a trance and having a hypnotic relationship may not be advised. There are no shoulds here and it's important to avoid the shoulds.

I suggest you use one of the best, not the very best hypnotic experience you've had. Simply because hypnosis like sex should not be a notion of always bigger and better. Not more orgasms, better orgasms and it's not a linear kind of thing. You need to give yourself the opportunity to meander and bring back different experiences. The harder you try the less you get back.

So, you can allow yourself to *let go and have what happens naturally happen*. You can take a stance of openness and curiosity and receptivity and you can go with the flow and flow as you glow. You can go ever *deeper down*. Deeper and deeper in a way that is right for you.

And certainly, *you can also adjust your position* however you'd like to so you can feel comfortable. A lot of times people start out with a certain posture or position and then want to change that and alter that, and that's fine. You certainly should give yourself permission, *a full permission* to do that.

And you know how you like to go down into hypnosis. But you don't always know the hypnotic *adventures* that you haven't yet had. What you don't know you will come to know, that what you'd **like to know you can be open to**. It's the only way to *learn something new*. You can go down into trance in a way that you respond and then you can add on or branch out while heading down.

And how is it that, you notice? What are the first signs that you have that you are going into trance? How do you know? I always go into trance when I do trance work. So, for me, it is the eyes open thing and a certain tunnel vision starts to develop. Others may see their first sign, a first hallmark of a deepening trance maybe a feeling of centeredness or relaxation or time distortion OR some sensory distortion. My voice may feel closer to you than you know that it can possibly be, which is off to the side and is participating but secondary. The subconscious influences can move ever more prominently into ascendance. Certainly, as we go into this experience you can feel free to, now or particularly later, if you feel an arm levitation to come over you, you can *allow your Dom* hand or non-dominate hand to rise up into the air. Naturally, easily, effortlessly as is the case with **sexual responding**. You simply set the stage and allow it to happen. So, one of the **adjustments in your positions** you can begin using now or later can be to have your hands in a position that would afford them the opportunity to effortlessly rise into the air.

As you allow yourself to wonder if that will happen in a couple of minutes or now or **toward the end or later back in the privacy of your room**, if they'll rise up into the air. You don't know, there's a lot of things that none of us know. That we want to begin to gain a notion of and be open and receptive to. Of course, I'm not simply going to recommend that each and every one of you do your own self-hypnosis. Being immersed in some of the experiences hypnotically have been the most positive experiences for you. You are welcome to utilize the induction that I often use in this and other circumstances like this.

In other groups, allowing yourself to go back, back in time. **To a time when you learned to do something that you didn't know that you could do.** You didn't know and it, maybe, was a little anxiety provoking at first, but then you began to see that ***this is so natural and something that so many people enjoy***. Many people enjoy learning the letters of the alphabet.

Can you remember that first day when you were in elementary school? When the teacher came in and put those letters up above the chalk board with little shiny tacks. Was it a black, blackboard, or a green board or a red blackboard? Was the teacher one of those really, really cool ones? Did and you know you had a pretty cool teacher when you realized there were a lot of different colors of chalk, and not just the white?

You can experience again now as fully as you wish, the letter A being written by the teacher on the blackboard. It's the first letter of the alphabet and you make it like this. There is a slanty line then make another slanty line that touches the first slanty line at the top. There is a connection there, and they touch, making a connection, and there is another connection that touches in the middle. Right across. Right across the middle and you write that first A, on the paper in front of you, it might have really wide lines and it looks different from the one that the adults use.

The paper looks almost as if it has chunks and little flakes and little chunks of wood in there and the pencil you are using can be especially big and thick and red. Sometimes it doesn't even have an eraser on the end. It's easier to hold because it is so big. ***It's nice to do things at first especially in a way that makes it easier to experience and to give you a positive experience***.

That's the role of the teacher, to foster a new experience in a way that's easier to get started; so that you ***have an experience of satisfaction***. So that you ***have a good first experience***. And then there is the letter B. B is the first letter of the word boy. There is a straight line and two curves. The two half circles that touch the straight line in the middle and you practice that. One row leads to another and you do it at home too as homework and you develop a sense of mastery.

When you get to the letter C you understand or begin to understand that it doesn't just get more difficult, some of them are easier. But none the less, you get to encounter and confront the issue. Is it the M that has 3 humps or two and is the N the same as a 3 turned on its side, upside down, reversed? Or how does that work? Once you get the letters going you know there are the numbers.

You learn your numbers and there are things that kids wonder like maybe everything we know we learned in kindergarten. But perhaps there's more opportunities to build on that. It's nice to have a sense of open awareness, in a sense, wondering. Is the 6 an upside down reversed 9? Or is it something different? What about the 2? If we take the 2 and turn it upside down and reverse it is it a 5, how can a 2 become a 5 and how can you allow that process and do it smoothly and play with the numbers. Over time you learn that you could do this and then cursive writing is introduced. You begin to wonder how I can attach all these words and letters together like the adults do. It seems so impossible at first, but *it happens and feels more and more natural. Naturally*. You learn something then that you may not know that you have learned before. Something that will serve you. Something that does serve you. That, just because an experience seems different or intimidating or you have doubts as to whether or not it's something for you. That you are going to be good at, it doesn't mean that you won't enjoy the process of trying and learning and seeing and discovering that yes, in fact, this is something that I can do. It's important to be discriminatingly brave. That's right, brave.

As you allow yourself to head back down deeper and deeper into hypnosis. I'd like to encourage you to visit some other things from back in time. You can time travel as a way of reminding yourself of some things you may have forgotten that you may need to know and what an affront to a person to think the best sexual experiences you ever had were or are over and relegated to the past for reasons that are not applicable and not good. Not enough people take an active approach to rekindling, rediscovering and moving forward with an erotic self and if you expect it to happen on its own, then it probably isn't going to happen. Or it's going to happen in a way that may or may not satisfy you; so it's helpful to be proactive at the helm, developing this facet. One part of yourself, the part that can energize, but is not a distraction, is something that informs and excites and energizes.

You can allow yourself to visit briefly or you can linger in certain key or important experiences from before and by asking yourself some certain solution focused discovery questions. When did I have the most fun in bed, and was it, in fact, that I was in bed? Who or what kind of person facilitates this and engenders this most easily in me, and under what conditions do I have really good intense orgasms?

How do I know that something new is something I would like to try? What about that time when you thought this was something that was , well that's something not for me. That's not my flavor. I don't care for that but you somehow managed to try it out a little bit only to discover that it really, really stimulated you. How can we organize, orchestrate, arrange sensible ways of finding out what it is that we don't think that we would enjoy, that could, in fact, be so fine and a pleasure to do?"

The person or group is now slowly brought out of hypnosis.

Dr. John H. Edgette

PART THREE: AFTER PLAY

CHAPTER 18
Each On Their Way

"Good sex is like good hypnosis - after both acts all parties warmly remember the experience and then casually part ways and fantasize about the next time" Dr. John H. Edgette

Having read this book, you now have learned how to help people who struggle with sexual issues, to resolve them. This will be a great contribution both to suffering clientele as well as prospective customers in need of help. You have acquired the tools to effect this positive change.

If you are new to hypnosis or a novice practitioner, there are a number of action steps to take while you simultaneously practice these techniques. The first is to consider joining a training group. Personal, one on one consultation with an expert is also a good idea. There are many options available, some at a very reasonable price. You are welcome to e-mail me (john@edgettetherapy.com) for recommendations regarding high quality training or supervision that will be individualized for you and your particular needs. Another thing to do is to practice on role playing volunteers, an action that will accomplish both the trying out of hypnotic work as well as sexual healing strategies.

If you are a journeyman or veteran hypnotist, you can go right to the action step of practicing on volunteers. If you are pretty confident of your abilities, then you can skip right to working with clients. It still is advisable to seek case consultation services. It is best if you work with someone who has expertise with both hypnosis and sexuality. Many consultants, such as myself, have an ability to work with people nationally or internationally via FaceTime or Zoom.

Whether working with volunteers or clients, it is very important to have them have their session with a friend or relative present. The accompanying person should be instructed to stay out of hypnosis and just watch. Likewise, I also recommend the subject audiotape the session, with the device for taping kept next to them. If they are using your device, you can send the recording to them electronically while they are in session.

The reason for these measures is to avoid any question of sexual improprieties. In hypnosis, as in any consultation regarding an issue, people can develop strong feelings toward the provider, and can act on them. Also, anything imagined in hypnosis is often thought to be absolutely real so these sessions could be fodder for false memory syndrome. These concerns are of even greater importance because here we are dealing with sexual issues.

In a similar vein, hypnotists should be extra professional at all times with the subject. This, for the reasons mentioned above but also because you are probably using the visceral, real life terms for sexuality that have been espoused by this book. Moreover, physical contact should be kept to a handshake at the start and finish of the session. This is no time to be a warm fuzzy or a hugger!

No matter where you are in your level of practice, it is always advisable to read about what you are doing. While there are not many good books out on hypnosis and sexuality per se, there are a plethora on hypnosis. Again, feel free to email me (john@edgettetherapy.com) for personalized recommendations. Anyone emailing me for this or other reasons will automatically be sent an advance chapter of one of my forthcoming books, Hypnotic Exotic Erotic (due out early 2021) or Hypnotic Erotic and Exotic: A Workbook. Heck, I will email you a chapter even if you just email me a simple question! I would enjoy hearing from you.

Whether hypnosis for sexual issues becomes a mainstay of your practice or a side hustle, you can make an epic difference in your clients lives with the tools you have been given in this book. Sex matters! Now go forth and provide sexual healing!

Dr. John H. Edgette

If you enjoyed this book please, please leave a 5-star review on Amazon or whatever platform you bought it from! This means a great deal to me and also inform other potential readers as to what to expect from the book! Thank you!

Hypnotic Erotic: A Practitioners Guide to Sexual Healing

Other books by Dr. John Edgette:

The Handbook of Hypnotic Phenomena in Psychotherapy (with J.S. Edgette).

Winning the Mind Game: Hypnosis and Sport Psychology (with Tim Rowan).

Forthcoming from Dr. John H. Edgette:

Hypnotic EXOTIC Erotic: A Practitioners Guide to Creating Sexual Adventurousness (Due out Late 2020)

Hypnotic Erotic And Exotic: A Workbook for Practitioners and Clients (due out early 2021)

Dr. John H. Edgette is available for practitioner or client consultation. He is also available for keynote speeches, workshops, seminars, or retreats. To schedule, email him at john@edgettetherapy.com.

John is also happy to answer any questions about the book or the issues discussed therein. He would also welcome all comments on this book. He can be reached at the above email.

www.ingramcontent.com/pod-product-compliance
Lightning Source LLC
Chambersburg PA
CBHW020256030426
42336CB00010B/797